Fat Weight Loss For Women In 2 Weeks
by Oswin Dacosta

Table of Contents

1. EFFECTIVE TIPS ON HOW TO REDUCE WEIGHT

Losing weight has always been a challenge for a good number of people. In as much as different people use different methods to lose weight, the common factors will always be regular exercise and a healthy diet. This will not only help you reduce weight but also maintain a healthy body. When all is said and done, the biggest challenge has always been consistency. Seen below are tips on how to reduce weight and keep it off.

1. Avoid processed foods.
Consuming too much of carbohydrates such as white bread, rice, with added sugar can result to excessive weight gain. In order to experience the opposite effect in this case being losing weight, your diet should consist of whole grains, whole meal bread and rice.

2. Set goals for motivation.
Coming up with short-term objectives such as having the need to fit into a specific outfit more often than not are not quite effective when compared to working towards becoming more confident or maintaining your health for the sake of your children. There are days when temptations may come your way or you may feel frustrated due to one reason or the other, instead of giving in focus on the numerous benefits you will enjoy as a result of the weight loss.

3. Steady weight loss.
Always work towards losing about a pound or two within a week in order to ensure that the process is done in a healthy manner. Drastic weight loss can negatively affect your body and mind. This will be evident as you begin to feel drained, sluggish and sick. When you drop too much weight too fast, you are simply losing water and muscle as opposed to fat.

4. Lifestyle change.
As you begin your weight loss journey, think of it as a lifestyle change as opposed to a temporary diet plan. The reason for this is because permanent weight loss can never be achieved by making use of quick fix diets. You should instead think of weight loss as a life time commitment. Making use of some of the popular diets available can actually give you the right foundation to start losing weight. However, long-term changes in regards to your lifestyle as well as the right food choices will definitely work best.

5. Tracking your progress.

Make use of the necessary tools to assist you in keeping track of your weight loss. Some examples include keeping a food journal. Here you can note down all the food that you eat on a daily basis. Having a weighing scale is also important as it will help you check on your weight and keep you motivated.

6. Support group.
Having social support is highly crucial. There are numerous support groups available for you to join. Here you will meet different people with whom you can share your experience with and learn from each other. Family and friends also play an important role when it comes to support.

Conclusion:
As earlier stated, you can easily lose weight but the problem for most people is maintaining it. However, by sticking to your lifestyle change and making use of the above tips you will be able to achieve your weight loss goals.

Please check out my websites: www.Losingbellyfatmission.com and www.achieveitforyou.com , and my book series "HOW TO GET ABS" and get in the best shape of your life:

http://www.amazon.com/dp/B00SSFWCPA

http://www.amazon.com/dp/B00QJJFS1C

http://www.amazon.com/dp/B00SX58DUI

Check out my other weight loss and Nutrition Books at:

http://www.amazon.com/dp/B00QH7DY4Y

http://www.amazon.com/dp/B00RVX3KY2

http://www.amazon.com/dp/B00QDHXN7Q

http://www.amazon.com/dp/B00PP8OZJ4

http://www.amazon.com/dp/B00PO0IQIO

2. Obesity is a major concern across the world today

The best way to fight obesity is to follow a strict healthy diet and a regular exercise regimen. A healthy weight loss diet should have fat burning foods. These foods help to burn excess body fats and suppress your appetite for unhealthy junk foods. Here are some foods which can burn body fat and speed up the metabolic rate.

Fat burning Foods

Water: Drinking plenty of water will speed up the metabolic rate and promote optimal bodily functions. So drink at least 8 glasses of water a day to burn off those extra calories.

Green Tea: Green tea contains chemicals, like Epigallocatechin gallate (EGCG) that helps burn fat and increases the metabolism. So including Green tea in your daily diet can help enhance your weight loss efforts.

Lean Protein: Including lean protein, like skinless chicken breasts, in your diet can significantly increase your metabolism. This is because protein digestion promotes cellular activities leading to fat burning and weight loss. The best sources of lean protein include lean chicken, egg whites, turkey breast and fish.

Complex High Fiber Carbs: Carbohydrates and fiber-rich foods are highly thermogenic and help fill you up so that you can go for longer periods without food. A combination of complex carbohydrates and lean protein promotes steady insulin production into the bloodstream and reduces insulin swings. The best complex high fiber carbs include brown rice, oatmeal, beans, non-starchy vegetables and whole grain breads.

Calcium: Calcium is not only vital for regulating hormonal activities in the body but it can also promote weight loss by burning fats. Rich sources of calcium include low-fat dairy products, almonds, leafy green vegetables and sesame seeds.

Vegetables: Eating high-fiber non-starchy veggies, such as cabbage, asparagus, broccoli, cauliflower, Brussels sprouts, spinach, endives, celery, peppers and tomatoes, can help boost metabolism since they have thermogenic properties and minimal effects on the insulin levels. By regulating your metabolism, these foods will help burn fat and calories.

Fruits: Including a variety of fruits in your diet will cleanse your body because it contains a lot of vitamins, fiber and water. The best fruit choices include apples, citrus fruit, cranberries, blueberries, strawberries, raspberries, melons, mangoes, pineapples and kiwi. Fruits that are rich in vitamin C, vitamin B12, vitamin E, phosphorus and potassium can boost your metabolism.

Spices: Hot spicy foods can temporarily boost your metabolism. For instance, the capsaicin compound present in peppers, stimulates the body to produce more stress hormones, speeding up your metabolic rate and increasing the body's ability to burn fats and calories. Best spices for fat burning include chilies, horseradish and cayenne.

Ginger and Garlic: Garlic and ginger raises the body temperature and stimulates the body's fat burning mechanism. So try to include them in your diet.

Essential Fatty Acids: Consuming Omega-3 essential fatty acids affects the levels of leptin in the body. Leptin is a fat hormone that influences the number of calories burnt or stored as fat. People with lower leptin levels will burn more calories compared to those with high leptin levels. The best omega 3 sources include tuna, salmon, sardines and lean white fish.

Including these foods in diet will fire up your metabolic rate and help you burn those excess fats. If you want to get the most out of these foods, combine them with a regular exercise regimen.

Please check out my websites: www.Losingbellyfatmission.com and www.achieveitforyou.com , and my book series "HOW TO GET ABS" and get in the best shape of your life:

http://www.amazon.com/dp/B00SSFWCPA

http://www.amazon.com/dp/B00QJJFS1C

http://www.amazon.com/dp/B00SX58DUI

Check out my other weight loss and Nutrition Books at:

http://www.amazon.com/dp/B00QH7DY4Y

http://www.amazon.com/dp/B00RVX3KY2

http://www.amazon.com/dp/B00QDHXN7Q

http://www.amazon.com/dp/B00PP8OZJ4

http://www.amazon.com/dp/B00PO0IQIO

3. How to Loose Body Fat

Loosing body fat is not easy; it requires patience, commitment, as well as making changes to personal daily habits. These are some of the methods that teach you how to loose body fat.

1. Reduce your Intake of Starchy Foods

Taking plenty of starchy foods at one sitting, such as bread, potatoes, and pasta among others provides the body with excess glycogen and energy stores. Once the body uses what it requires, the excess amount is stored as fat. Starchy foods are essential for the body, but you should reduce their intake when trying to loose body fat.

2. Exercise

Once you decide to loose body fat, it is important that you develop an exercise routine and follow it. For example, you can exercise in a moderate manner through weights and aerobics since these increases the chances of losing body fat. Furthermore, when starting out, it is important that you begin with low-intensity weight and aerobic training to avoid placing the body through unnecessary stress.

3. Drink Plenty of Water

Drinking plenty of water makes you full, and assists in reducing the amount of food that you eat. It is advisable to take one ounce of water for every two pounds of body weight every day. You will be surprised at how much body fat you can lose by following this method.

4. Reduce your Sugar Intake

Consuming small amounts of sugar immediately after an exercise session replenishes liver and muscle glycogen stores. However, any excess amount of sugar taken afterwards is stored as fat in the body. If you decide to take beverages afterwards, it is advisable to take diet soda, water with juice, tea, or coffee. That will ensure that no fat is stored in the body, taking you closer to accomplishing your goal of losing body fat.

5. Space your Meals

In the process of losing body fat, it is advisable that you take small meals, and give them a space of two to three hours. Every meal should be balanced with proteins and carbohydrates. Skipping a meal is not good, in the process of losing body fat. Therefore, you should eat often and healthy.

6. Eat a Diet Rich in Fiber

According to research, fiber decreases the calorie and insulin levels. In addition, fiber assists in water absorption, and fills your stomach, reducing the hunger discomfort that may come your way.

7. Drink Some Milk

Studies have shown that taking calcium through dairy products, such as fat free cheese, as well as yoghurt can assist in reducing the absorption of fat from other sources of food.

8. Stay away From Junk Food

Junk food is any food that gives plenty of calories to the body. Some of the junk foods that you should avoid include sweets, and French fries. However, other foods such as hamburgers and pizza, which many consider junk food, offer nutritional benefits to the body. Eating these foods, once in a while when on a diet, can be helpful.

There you have it. Those are eight ways that will assist you in losing your body fat. Follow them, and you will be amazed at the positive results that they can provide.

4. What Is The Best Belly Fat Diet?

Losing weight especially in the abdominal area is one of the most challenging things when it comes to fitness, and that is why there have been countless products out there focusing on this specific problem. If you want to get rid of your belly fat, then there are a couple things you should know. No matter how many personal trainers you have, if you don't follow a healthy diet, you will never achieve the body you want. Fitness and having a slim physique is 20% exercise and 80% your diet, and so if you really want that perfect flat stomach, make sure to follow a clean diet.

What Is The Best Belly Fat Diet?

There really is no specific diet that you can do to burn belly fat, as there are many diets that work quite well. Unfortunately, most fad diets that are effective don't actually offer long term results. When you go on a crash diet and lose the weight you want, you are very much likely to just gain the weight back, because the diet you followed isn't one you can continue for a long period of time. The best way to lose belly fat is by following a healthy diet that you can continuously do for the rest of your life. One of the best ways to consistently follow a healthy diet is to just portion control. It is completely okay to have a bit of that pizza you've been dying to eat as long as you don't eat too much of it. The more you deprive yourself, the harder it will be to continue eating healthy. Aside from portion control, it is also important to choose the right foods to burn the belly fat. The fat that is produced within the abdominal area is very stubborn and difficult to burn, but certain foods have been shown to counteract that toughness to soften it and tighten it completely.

Top Foods That Burn Belly Fat

A few of the best foods for stomach fat include young coconut, egg, kale, oatmeal, turmeric, non-fat yogurt, mango, broccoli, and salmon. As you can see these foods are not processed packaged foods you find in the chips aisle at your grocery store. The key to losing fat is to always buy food that you would easily find thousands of years ago. Try your best to avoid fast, junk, and frozen foods, as they all happen to be some of the worst things your body to have. The main ingredient you want to look for in your food is protein, because protein helps to speed up the metabolism and produce muscle in your body. The main ingredient you want to avoid is sugar, as sugar just turns into pure fat in the body and is the hardest type of fat to burn.

Your diet should be balanced from the protein to the sodium, and from the sugar to the calcium. Be a smart eater and always remember to chew as much as possible to really dissolve the food in your mouth before it goes into your body.

5. How to effectively loose weight in just two weeks

If a time span of two weeks is what you have so as to shed some pounds from your body, you can definitely wonder how much you can loose in that period of time. However, this is a very easy undertaking that only calls for a strategic plan, firm commitment and a great extent of willpower. In most cases, the results achieved will be different among various people due to the various genetic variations in our bodies. Weight loss in 2 weeks is not an easy task but is highly possible if done in the appropriate ways.

For a 2 weeks weight loss program to be effective and fruitful, there are some essential tips that must be adhered to. First, before going on any weight loss program, it is worth noting that no miracles or magic can help you loose weight over night. Many people opt to use weight loss pill as a weight loss mechanism in a motive to avoid the gym but as a matter of fact, using such pills can only lead to loss of money and not weight. This therefore means that for effective weight loss, frequent body exercises have to be done.

When you think of weight loss in 2 weeks, it is also important to consider your diet and eating habits during the time period. When on such a weight loss program, foods such as chips, soda and other junk foods should be avoided since they contain ingredients with high fat levels. When on such a weight loss program, it is important to take caution on the kind of diet you take and important of all, a lot of water should be consumed. By avoiding junk foods, it becomes easier for you to take part in weight loss exercises which increase the body's metabolic rate. The perfect diet for an individual in a 2 weeks weight loss program should have more of vegetables, legumes, fluids and lean proteins. carbohydrates and fats should be avoided as much as possible. By using a comfortable, effective and sensible diet, it is not a surprise to loose ten pounds in a fortnight. However, when on a diet, it is advisable not to starve your body by skipping some meals.

If you are to effectively loose weight in two weeks, you must be ready to increase the physical activities of the body by engaging in exercises. In most cases, it is advisable to have a thirty-minutes period on a daily basis to exercise your body. Exercise can be in the form of a light jog, a walk, cycling, dancing or even an aerobics class attendance. This way, two weeks will even be more than enough for you to lose ten pounds. So as to avoid engaging in very strenuous exercises, people on a 2 weeks weight loss plan are advised to use weight loss pills as supplements for the exercises. With proper commitment and willingness to shed some body calories, weight loss in two weeks can be easily achieved without much struggle and hustle.

6. Easiest weight loss plan, easiest way to loose weight

Millions of people in the world are facing the challenge of having to deal with weight loss. They try to find easy and safe ways that they can use to lose weight. One of the fundamental requirements when you need a plan to lose weight safely is to try and get an easy weight loss plan, which you can use to help you lose your weight faster, easily and most important safely. Researchers in weight loss have found out that people who employ easy methods to try and lose weight find the process to be fun and record over 90% success rate compared to those who employ complicated and hard weight loss plans.

When a person is overweight, it does not only make them feel uncomfortable, but also pose severe health problems. It is at times hard to being the process of weight loss. However, with an easy weight loss plan in place; it is highly likely that you will begin to record positive results within a very short period of time.

Features of easy weight loss plan/ Easy ways to lose weight.

One of the key features of any weight loss plan is that it should include a good exercise program. However, the difference is that for an easy weight loss plan the exercise plan should not be extremely intense such that the individual that is trying to lose weight finds it a punishment. The exercise program should be full of fun, with 3 day workout program every week at minimum.

Fruits and vegetables without any doubt are essential part of an easy weight loss plan. This is because they are usually loaded with lots of fiber, vitamins as well as antioxidants making them important for weight loss purpose.

An important feature of weight loss plan is the proportions of different types of things that should be in your diet menu. You do not need to starve yourself so that you can lose weight. In fact dieting is a misunderstood concept. What is important is that you have an easy and proper diet plan on what you are going to eat on each day of the week. You can have something like this;

Day1

Breakfast
1 cup of Milk and 1 orange.

Lunch
1 whole grain peta bread and 1 cup of skim milk.

Dinner

Half cup of cooked brown rice and yellow beans, ? piece of banana

Day 2

Breakfast

? cup of some skim milk
? piece of banana.

Lunch

1/2 piece of pineapple
A slice of reduced-Calorie Oatmeal Bran Bread

Dinner

? cup Cooked Quinoa and 1 Nectarine.
? cup of fresh blended fruit juice.

You are expected to observe such a diet plan for seven days a week each day planned differently with foods that are likely to support your weight loss goals.

In you diet plan ensure that you eat at least five to seven small meals each day. Instead of just having to stuff yourself for just 2 to 3 times a day, this helps to keep blood sugar levels in balance. Secondly, avoid processed and fast foods since they have high sodium and fat content.

It is important to remember that an easy weight loss plan should not include sugary drinks, instead it is expected that a lot of water will be part of the diet which should be at least eight glasses each day. This keeps the body hydrated making you feel full through out the day.

Document by keeping records of your food intake so that you are able to know the number of calories you ingest daily. Do not also be too hard on yourself. Make the whole experience in your weight loss plan fun by rewarding yourself randomly.

7. Why Staying Healthy So Is Important?

If you ask a healthcare expert whether it's important to stay healthy, he will undoubtedly answer with a yes. However, if you ask why staying healthy is important, you might notice a pause. A better understanding of why staying healthy is important gives you greater motivation and encouragement to focus on a healthy diet and exercise regime. In addition to this, if you understand the numerous benefits of staying healthy, you can also motivate your loved ones and friends to follow a healthy lifestyle.

Survival of the Fittest

Unless you participate in dangerous activities on a regular basis, the most important tip to increase your chances at a long life is to remain healthy and fit. According to the CDC, a person who remains physically active for 7 hours per week is about 40% less likely to suffer health problems or die early than a person who's physically active for less than half an hour per week. When you remain healthy, it reduces your chances of suffering from stroke, heart disease, type 2 diabetes, osteoporosis, high blood pressure and different kinds of cancer.

Declaration of Independence

In addition to living a longer life, staying healthy gives you a better quality of life. It gives you a good chance to remain independent throughout your life. When you consume a healthy diet and exercise regularly, you stay in good shape. This provides you with more energy to perform routine tasks at home and work. This increases your productivity and efficiency. Thus, it's more likely that you will have good energy to spare when your daily work is over. If you stay healthy as you get older, you reduce the risk of falling. In simple terms, a healthy person is not only at reduced risk for various diseases, but also less likely to get injured.

Use Your Head

According to healthcare experts, the human body and mind are connected to each other. Healthcare professionals understand this connection, and recommend a healthy diet and workout regime. According to most fitness experts and nutritionists, staying fit and healthy reduces the risk of depression. It helps you maintain a fit and healthy brain. Just like muscles, the brain is a physical construction. Therefore, it also declines with age. Just like experience keeps your body healthy, proper health can make sure your brain remains productive and prevents age related effects.

An Apple a Day

Last but not the least, staying healthy also offers monetary benefits. It's quite obvious that a healthy and fit individual does not have to spend a lot of money on healthcare. Unlike an unfit person, a healthy person does not have to visit doctors frequently. Being healthy not only helps you save money in the present, but also the future. According to a study conducted in 2012, the healthcare costs of more than 20,000 men and women was taken into account. The study concluded that healthy people see a reduction of about 40% in medical costs in later years of life. It's important to focus on a healthy diet and regular workouts to stay healthy, and enjoy all these benefits throughout your life.

8. Women's Versus Men's Metabolism

Everyone knows that losing weight and maintaining it is not an easy task. Women have to face an even tougher task as the vast majority of weight loss researches have been done on men. There is no denying that women's body differ from men's in a lot of ways, but metabolism is one of the factor concerns that determine the results or exercise response on one's body and this factor plays significantly different role at different levels in both the genders.

Women's V/S Men's Metabolism - Facts You Should Know!

At Rest, Women Burn Carbs More Than Men, But Less Fat

Research suggests that women have a low percentage of DHA due to low intake of omega-3s. This can lead to significant weight gain at the time of pregnancy. Apparently, women have greater fat storage, which also contributes to high body fat percentage. Once a young woman is able to reproduce, her body begins storing fat around thighs and the hips to prepare the body to carry a baby. This leads to significant weight gain. Regardless of what your fitness goals are, get adequate DHA in your diet to get balanced ratio of omega-3 fats to omega-6 fats. This makes your body metabolically flexible.

Women and Men Burn And Store Body Fat Differently

A Woman's body is said to rely on fat for fuel and at a high degree than a man. This is the reason why it is very important for women to exercise on a daily basis. Women lose fat from the upper body first, and tend to have a difficult time losing from the lower body. Also, women store fat right below the skin, while men have more visceral fat which is metabolically active. Scientists suggest that indulging in higher intensity of resistance exercise can help stimulate the release the body fat from fat cells.

Stress Affects Women's Metabolism That Inhibits Fat Loss

Stress can affect fat loss abilities for everyone, but certain kinds of stress can be more harmful to women in comparison to men. It is necessary to find some kind of stress management strategies that could work for you. Meditation, psychological therapy, yoga, etc. are good options to consider. Stress leads to persistent secretion of cortisol, which increases blood sugar to help your body to fight the stressful situation.

Intermittent Fasting And Less Calorie Intake Is Detrimental for Women, But Beneficial for Men

Intermittent fasting (IF) and restricted calorie intake have become a good example for weight loss, but it does not work for women. Stress on body system negatively affects a woman's metabolism as compared to men. Intermittent fasting and calorie deficit diet are metabolically beneficial for men, allowing them to lose more fat, improving disease risk factors and reducing inflammation. However, researches have shown that fasting is harmful for women. So while it allows men to lose weight, women gain it. Women should avoid relying on calorie restriction for weight loss. They should strictly stay away from fasting and detoxification diets. If you provide your body with enough energy, balanced fat, protein and carbs, your hormones will get in balance, your stress will reduce and your body will start losing fat.

9. Women Tips on How to Lose Fat Weight without Straining Yourself

Majority of women around the globe are searching for a solution on how to slash down those extra fat weight quickly and get back a nice shape. This is as a result of the rising awareness of the serious risk of being overweight. Nowadays people are aware that having too much fat can lead to many deadly diseases such as hypertension, heart diseases, diabetes and arthritis.

Ladies are going for ads that claim to have a weight loss program designed for them. Women torture themselves with these claims since they do not give excellent result as expected. But they do not have worry anymore as there are effective ways for women to lose fat weight fast and safe. Get that body shape and size you wish for without going physically broke doing it.

Here are some tips meant for women on how to successfully lose fat weight.

Motivation: You cannot attain your goal of losing fat weight without motivation. This is a very powerful reason to keep on changing your bad habit to good for fat loss. Have your own motivation not another person's. Discover things that make you ardent like love .By loving someone else it means you can go extra miles to satisfy their need and by making others happy you are also feeding your soul with energetic vibes. Guide that feeling to become your weight loss motivator for there is no better motivator than the other. And each time your bad or old habits call, you will have a good reminder of why you decided to get trim and loose weight.

Healthy eating habit: Try eating the premium of everything. Consume meals prepared with totally healthy oils and fresh constituent. Different herbs, vegetables cheese and seasonings are good choices of food for weight lose. You will even start feeling better nearly immediately. Majority of overweight women are surprisingly undernourished. They feel unhealthy and lack alertness due to their bodies being deficiency of vitamins and minerals. But eating meals prepared out of fresh constituents can actually help by correcting this imbalance and in turn you will easily lose fat weight unknowingly.

Moderate exercise: The easiest way to lose weight through exercising is by having a walk. Since most deskbound women give up before having met the desired result. You can avoid going to the nearest markets or take a walk from work to avoid introducing this program among your plans or straining yourself by walking then going to carry out other duties. Walk to any extent provided that you are enjoying the habit and listening to your body. By doing this you will be stress free, sleeping better and eventually lose weight permanently.

Aim: Do not strain yourself too much to get a celebrity body shape since a celebrity lives a comfortable and less taxing life not like a common woman that works for 10 hours or more daily. Acknowledge the difference between both lifestyles and begin making a few changes everyday. For instance, eat more fruit during meals and in a couple of days you will witness weight shift and fat loss taking place.

Put these tips in to practice and you will surely stand a chance of gaining more. Take a step toward achieving a better body size and shape. Also maintain your perfect weight and live healthy life by losing weight and fat.

10. Nutrition and Health

Nutrition and health go hand in hand because nutrition plays an integral role in the normal growth of the human body and its functions. Nutrients provide the cells with the energy to run the body. Lack of proper nutrients exposes the body to various diseases and conditions. On the same note, unhealthy eating habits can lead to obesity which is equally dangerous to the body. A person suffering from obesity has a high risk of developing a number of diseases such as stroke, heart dysfunction, diabetes, cancer and other heart related diseases. So to avoid these diseases, you should make healthy food choices that would guarantee a healthy heart.

Diet for healthy heart

General dietary tips for keeping the heart healthy includes eating a well-balanced diet with less fat and sugar. You can change your dieting habits by including the following heart healthy foods:

- Salmon is rich in omega-3 essential fatty acids that reduce the risks of both inflammation and blood clots, thereby protecting the heart. These fats also help to maintain your cholesterol at healthy levels. Eating salmon, tuna, herring and sardines at least twice per week will go a long way in keeping your heart healthy.

- Olive oil is an essential part of Mediterranean diet which lowers LDL cholesterol levels, thereby reducing the risk of heart disease. You can consume olive oil by using it for cooking, or by making a dip for whole grain bread.

- Oats are rich in a soluble fiber known as beta glucan that can help reduce the levels of LDL cholesterol and total cholesterol. Soluble fiber is also important in keeping the digestive system healthy. Enjoy oatmeal with plenty of walnuts and strawberries for breakfast.

- Apples are rich in a phytochemical known as quercetin which has anti-inflammatory properties and may also prevent blood clots. Apples are good sources of vitamins and fiber and also come in many delicious varieties.

- Almonds contain vitamin E, healthy oils and other essential substances that would help control your cholesterol levels. Almonds are also rich in fiber and protein. Almonds can make an excellent snack on their own.

- Whole grains contain fiber and vitamins that will help to keep the heart healthy. You can consume it in the form of whole grain bread or whole grain pasta.

- Green leafy vegetables are rich in Vitamin E and folate, which helps to reduce homocysteine levels. Green leafy vegetables can also help to improve memory. Use fresh leaves of spinach or other greens to make your favorite salad.

- Tomatoes contain lycopene and vitamins, which play a role in reducing heart disease risk. Add thick tomato slices to salads and sandwiches or enjoy tomato sauce on pasta.

- Soy protein can prevent heart diseases by reducing the intake of saturated fat, which makes it a great protein substitute for red meat. You can consume soy protein by adding soy milk to your morning cereal.

So, plan your daily diet and pack it with as much healthy foods as possible. If you follow these healthy food tips, you will soon notice a considerable difference in your heart health and overall health. You may also check out my free video on weight loss at www.achieveitforyou.com.

Please check out my websites: www.Losingbellyfatmission.com and www.achieveitforyou.com , and my book series "HOW TO GET ABS" and get in the best shape of your life:

http://www.amazon.com/dp/B00SSFWCPA

http://www.amazon.com/dp/B00QJJFS1C

http://www.amazon.com/dp/B00SX58DUI

Check out my other weight loss and Nutrition Books at:

http://www.amazon.com/dp/B00QH7DY4Y

http://www.amazon.com/dp/B00RVX3KY2

http://www.amazon.com/dp/B00QDHXN7Q

http://www.amazon.com/dp/B00PP8OZJ4

http://www.amazon.com/dp/B00PO0IQIO